An Overview of
HEADACHES

An Overview of HEADACHES

V Natarajan
MD DM(Neurology) FRCP(Edinburgh) FAAN FIAN FIMSA
Former Professor and Head of Neurology
Institute of Neurology
Madras Medical College
Professor Emeritus
The Tamil Nadu Dr MGR Medical University
Chennai, Tamil Nadu, India

K Mugundhan
MD DM(Neurology) FRCP(Glasgow) FRCP(London) FRCP(Ireland)
FRCP(Edinburgh) FACP(USA) FICP FICCDMD FIMSA
Professor and Head of Neurology
Stanley Medical College
Chennai, Tamil Nadu, India

Forewords
Girish Mathur
Jyotirmoy Pal

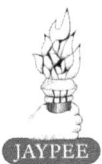

JAYPEE BROTHERS MEDICAL PUBLISHERS
The Health Sciences Publisher
New Delhi | London

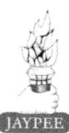 **Jaypee Brothers Medical Publishers (P) Ltd**

Headquarters
EMCA House
23/23-B, Ansari Road, Daryaganj
New Delhi 110 002, India
Landline: +91-11-23272143, +91-11-23272703
+91-11-23282021, +91-11-23245672
E-mail: jaypee@jaypeebrothers.com

Corporate Office
Jaypee Brothers Medical Publishers (P) Ltd.
4838/24, Ansari Road, Daryaganj
New Delhi 110 002, India
Phone: +91-11-43574357
Fax: +91-11-43574314
E-mail: jaypee@jaypeebrothers.com

Overseas Office
JP Medical Ltd.
83, Victoria Street, London
SW1H 0HW (UK)
Phone: +44-20 3170 8910
Fax: +44(0)20 3008 6180
E-mail: info@jpmedpub.com

EU GPSR Authorised Representative
LOGOS EUROPE, 9 rue Nicolas Poussin
17000, LA ROCHELLE, France
Phone: +33 (0) 6 67 93 73 78
Email: Contact@logos europe.eu

Website: www.jaypeebrothers.com
Website: www.jaypeedigital.com

© 2024, Jaypee Brothers Medical Publishers

The views and opinions expressed in this book are solely those of the original contributor(s)/author(s) and do not necessarily represent those of editor(s) or publisher of the book.

All rights reserved. No part of this publication may be reproduced, stored or transmitted in any form or by any means, electronic, mechanical, photocopying, recording or otherwise, without the prior permission in writing of the publishers.

All brand names and product names used in this book are trade names, service marks, trademarks or registered trademarks of their respective owners. The publisher is not associated with any product or vendor mentioned in this book.

Medical knowledge and practice change constantly. This book is designed to provide accurate, authoritative information about the subject matter in question. However, readers are advised to check the most current information available on procedures included and check information from the manufacturer of each product to be administered, to verify the recommended dose, formula, method and duration of administration, adverse effects and contraindications. It is the responsibility of the practitioner to take all appropriate safety precautions. Neither the publisher nor the author(s)/editor(s) assume any liability for any injury and/or damage to persons or property arising from or related to use of material in this book.

This book is sold on the understanding that the publisher is not engaged in providing professional medical services. If such advice or services are required, the services of a competent medical professional should be sought.

Every effort has been made where necessary to contact holders of copyright to obtain permission to reproduce copyright material. If any have been inadvertently overlooked, the publisher will be pleased to make the necessary arrangements at the first opportunity.

Inquiries for bulk sales may be solicited at: jaypee@jaypeebrothers.com

An Overview of Headaches / V Natarajan, K Mugundhan

First Edition: **2024**

ISBN: 978-93-5696-596-6

Foreword

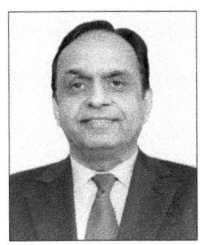

Girish Mathur MD FICP FACP FRCP(London, Glasgow, Edinburgh)
FIACM FRSSDI Fellow Diabetes India
President, Association of Physicians of India

I am delighted to write foreword for the handbook on *"An Overview of Headaches"* by esteemed Neurophysicians Dr V Natarajan and Dr K Mugundhan.

Headache is one of the most common symptom with which a patient visits a doctor and at times may pose as one of the most perplexing of all clinical problems.

It may not always be possible to unravel the cause of headache because in many cases it can be because of a simpler etiology but a thorough and methodical approach is needed to reach to a diagnosis to rule out underlying serious disorders.

It is heartening to note that the authors of this handbook have taken utmost care to narrate the whole spectrum of headaches in most simplified manner.

I congratulate Dr V Natarajan and Dr K Mugundhan to undertake the task of writing this handbook, which I am sure will prove to be of immense use to common practicing physicians.

Foreword

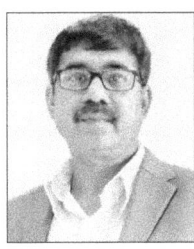

Jyotirmoy Pal MD FRCP(London, Glasgow, Edinburgh) FICP FACP WHO Fellow
Dean, Indian College of Physicians

I congratulate Dr V Natarajan and Dr K Mugundhan for presenting this book on *"An Overview of Headaches"*, which is a practical guide to approach this very common ailment. I am sure this book will be very helpful to physicians in their daily practice. The cases given will be helpful for analytical decision making. It will also highlight the knowledge as to identify red flag signs for timely referral and prompt intervention.

Best wishes for the future.

Preface

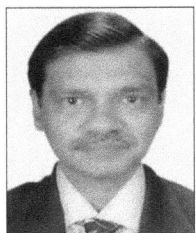

V Natarajan MD DM(Neurology)
FRCP(Edinburgh) FAAN FIAN FIMSA
Former Professor and Head of Neurology
Institute of Neurology
Madras Medical College
Professor Emeritus
The Tamil Nadu Dr MGR Medical University
Chennai, Tamil Nadu, India

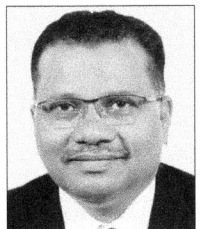

K Mugundhan MD DM(Neurology)
FRCP(Glasgow) FRCP(London) FRCP(Ireland)
FRCP(Edinburgh) FACP(USA) FICP FICCDMD
FIMSA
Professor and Head of Neurology
Stanley Medical College
Chennai, Tamil Nadu, India

This is only *"An Overview of Headaches"* as it is impossible to cover extensively in a monogram.

This monogram will cover the practical aspects of how to proceed when facing a patient having a headache and will not be dealing much on detailing of studies or pathomechanics.

The aim is to help practitioners to know and identify some of the common headache presentations to enable them to appropriately choose which patient to investigate and, or refer the patient to a specialist or a higher center of further management.

The case vignettes provided by my colleagues highlight the clinical presentation of some of the causes of secondary headaches.

V Natarajan

K Mugundhan

Acknowledgments

We are extremely grateful to Dr Girish Mathur, President, API, and Dr Jyotirmoy Pal, Dean, ICP for their kind words in the Foreword.

We are deeply indebted to our teachers Professor K Jaganathan and Professor G Arjun Das, Former Professors, Institute of Neurology, Chennai, whose inspiration and guidance have been our biggest strength and source of energy.

We are grateful to our colleagues Dr PR Sowmini and Dr M Sathish Kumar Assistant Professors of Neurology, Stanley Medical College, Chennai, Tamil Nadu, India, for their help in writing this book.

We would like to thank all our patients who were true sources of inspiration behind this book.

We would also like to extend our gratitude to our family members.

We especially appreciate the constant support and encouragement of Shri Jitendar P Vij (Group Chairman) and Mr Ankit Vij (Managing Director) of M/s Jaypee Brothers Medical Publishers (P) Ltd, New Delhi, India, in publishing the book and also their associates, particularly Ms Chetna Malhotra (Senior Director—Professional Publishing, Marketing, and Business Development), and Ms Asmi Bharati (Development Editor), who have been prompt, efficient, and most helpful.

Contents

CHAPTER 1:   Introduction — 1

CHAPTER 2:   Types — 2

CHAPTER 3:   Approach — 3

CHAPTER 4:   History — 5

CHAPTER 5:   Neurological Examination — 6

CHAPTER 6:   The Red Flags Go Under the Rubric SNOOP — 7

CHAPTER 7:   Imaging — 8

CHAPTER 8:   Primary Headaches — 10

CHAPTER 9:   Migraine — 11

CHAPTER 10: Phases of Migraine — 12

CHAPTER 11: Migraine Features — 13

CHAPTER 12: Pathophysiology of Migraine — 14

CHAPTER 13: Treatment of Migraine — 15

CHAPTER 14: Migraine Prevention — 17

CHAPTER 15: Tension-type Headaches — 18

CHAPTER 16: Treatment of Tension-type Headache — 19

CHAPTER 17: Trigeminal Autonomic Cephalgias — 20

CHAPTER 18: Other Primary Headaches — 23

CHAPTER 19: Secondary Headaches — 26

CHAPTER 20: Neuralgias — 29

CHAPTER 21: **Headaches and Sinus Disease**   31

CHAPTER 22: **Challenges**   33

CHAPTER 23: **Case Discussion**   35

Index   41

CHAPTER 1

Introduction

Headache is caused by pain sensitive structures within the cranium and also by those outside the cranium. It should be realized that brain as such is insensitive to pain. The intracranial structures which are sensitive to pain are the blood vessels namely the arteries, veins and the venous sinuses, and the dura mater covering the brain.

The extracranial structures that are sensitive to pain are the paranasal sinuses, the eyes and the orbits, the ears including the tympanic membrane, teeth, salivary glands, and the temporomandibular joints, cervical roots, and blood vessels.

CHAPTER 2

Types

There are innumerable types of headaches approximately > 300 types which for ease of convenience and practicality can be classified into primary headaches and secondary headaches.

The primary headaches are much more common constituting about 90% of the headaches and are so called as there are no underlying structural or metabolic abnormalities causing the headaches.

Secondary headaches are due to an underlying abnormality which may be structural or metabolic and constitute approximately 10% of the headaches. These structural abnormalities can be within the cranium like vascular causes of aneurysms or arteriovenous malformations which result in bleeding inside the brain or in the space between the coverings or outside as with subarachnoid hemorrhage or subdural hemorrhage usually following a trauma to the head.

Other vascular causes include thrombosis of cerebral venous sinus thrombosis (CVST) and less commonly of the arteries, and reversible cerebral vasoconstriction syndrome (RCVS) apart from dissection of cranial blood vessels.

The nonvascular structural abnormalities would include tumors and infections—meningitis and abscess.

The metabolic causes giving rise to rather persistent headaches would include carbon dioxide retention, carbon monoxide poisoning, and hypoxia.

CHAPTER **3**

Approach

HISTORY AND CLINICAL EXAMINATION

The first and the most important step would be to take a detailed history of the headaches and do an appropriate neurological examination.

The history would be most crucial in deciding whether the headache is primary or secondary with assistance from the neurological examination. Abnormal findings on examination would certainly point to a secondary headache and the next step would be to try and ascertain the cause.

The approach to headache should be to identify whether it is primary or secondary as the management varies according to that. If considered secondary, the underlying cause should be found out and appropriately treated **(Flowchart 1)**.

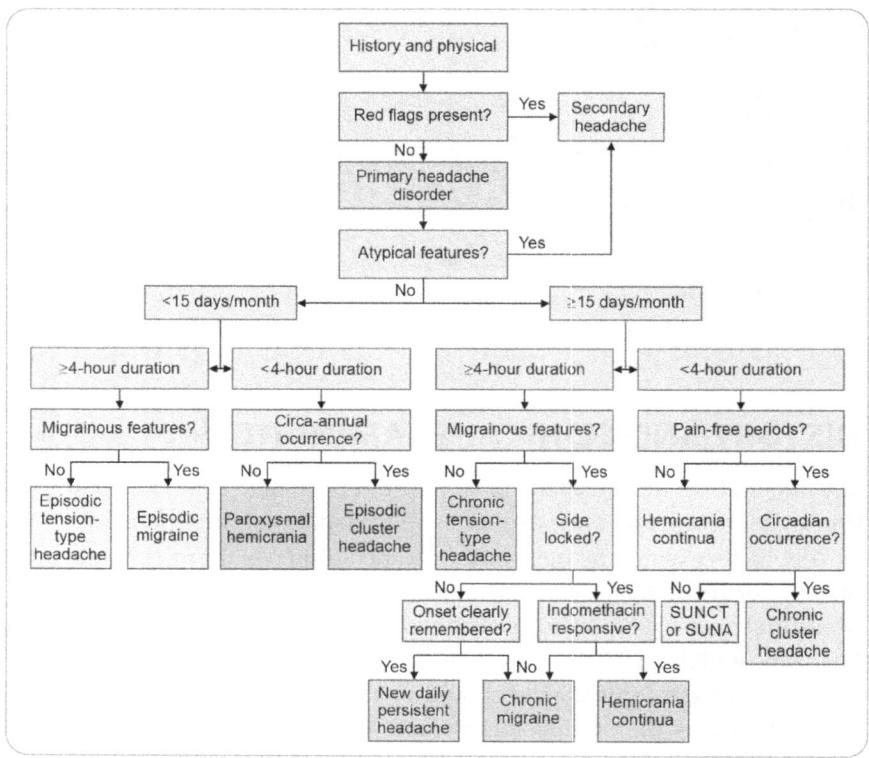

FLOWCHART 1: Approach to headache.
(SUNA: short-lasting unilateral neuralgiform headache attacks with cranial autonomic symptoms; SUNCT: short-lasting unilateral neuralgiform headache with conjunctival injection and tearing)

CHAPTER 4

History

The following details should be found out from the history:
- Is the headache recurrent and episodic?
- What is the frequency, severity, duration, and location of the headache?
- Is the headache always similar or are there different types of pain?
- What is the nature of the pain? Throbbing, a tight sensation around the head or as though a weight is placed over the head or lancinating, stabbing?
- What are the associated features with the headaches? Nausea, vomiting, photophobia, osmophobia, redness of the eyes, tearing, swelling of the periorbital region, and narrowing of the palpebral fissures?
- Further details to be obtained include details of the triggers for the headaches such as:
  - Lack of sleep
  - Exposure to sun
  - Stress
  - Periods
  - Head bath
  - Long distance travel
  - Hunger
  - Change in weather
  - Relation to neck position in sleep
- Whether there is a periodicity to the occurrence of the headaches and does they occur in clusters?
- Are there additional features such as vertigo, tinnitus, confusion, altered sensorium, seizures, and visual obscurations?
- Do visual, sensory, and speech auras occur?

CHAPTER **5**

Neurological Examination

The neurological examination of the patient with headaches should include examination of the visual acuity, visual field, ocular fundi, and look out for focal deficits **(Fig. 1)**.

Focal deficits identification should include examination of the motor system for weakness of limbs or unsteadiness and examination of language functions in the form of speech defects.

Sensory examination also needs to be done as migraine patients could report sensory symptoms which would not be associated with abnormalities on examination as it would represent a sensory aura of migraine. However, if sensory examination is abnormal it would indicate that the headache is not primary and a search for an underlying cause has to be done as with other abnormalities detected on neurological examination.

A normal neurological examination would suggest a primary headache disorder with certain caveats which are considered as red flags.

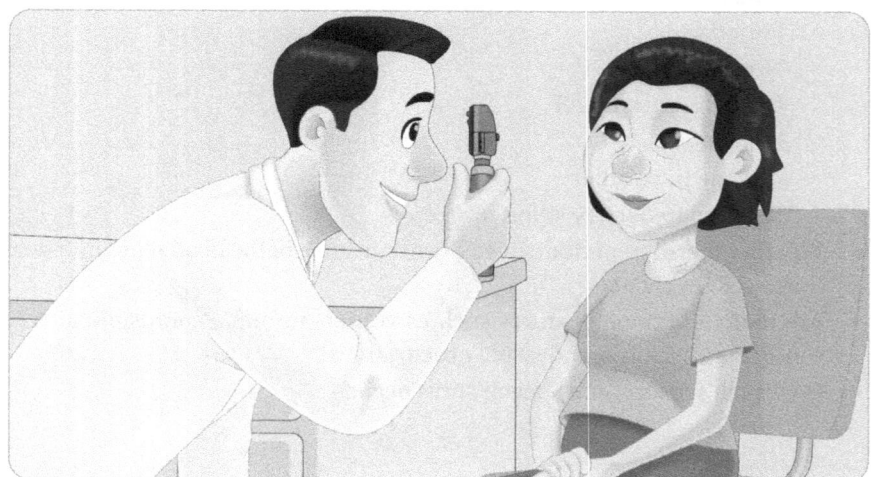

FIG. 1: Examination of visual acuity, visual field, and ocular fundi.

CHAPTER 6

The Red Flags Go Under the Rubric SNOOP

There are a number of red flags, the mnemonic for which is *SNOOP*:

S—systemic symptoms such as fever, weight loss, secondary headache risk factors like human immunodeficiency virus (HIV), cancer, pregnancy, and postpartum period.

N—neurologic symptoms or signs namely confusion, altered sensorium, or focal neurologic deficits.

O—onset being sudden or abrupt in a split second like a thunderclap.

O—older age and new onset or progressive headache in a person with age >50 years as with giant cell arteritis.

P—no history of previous headache or headache which is progressive in intensity. A first headache or a headache which has changed its pattern, with regards its frequency, severity, or clinical features.

CHAPTER 7

Imaging

All patients who show abnormal findings on examination or those whose headache history is not consistent with one of the primary headaches by the description given need imaging of the brain to exclude a structural abnormality **(Fig. 1)**.

The best mode of imaging would be to do magnetic resonance imaging (MRI) as that is superior to computerized tomography (CT) scan of the head, especially in identifying following conditions:
- Vascular disorders such as saccular aneurysms, arteriovenous malformations (AVMs), subarachnoid hemorrhage (SAH), carotid or vertebral

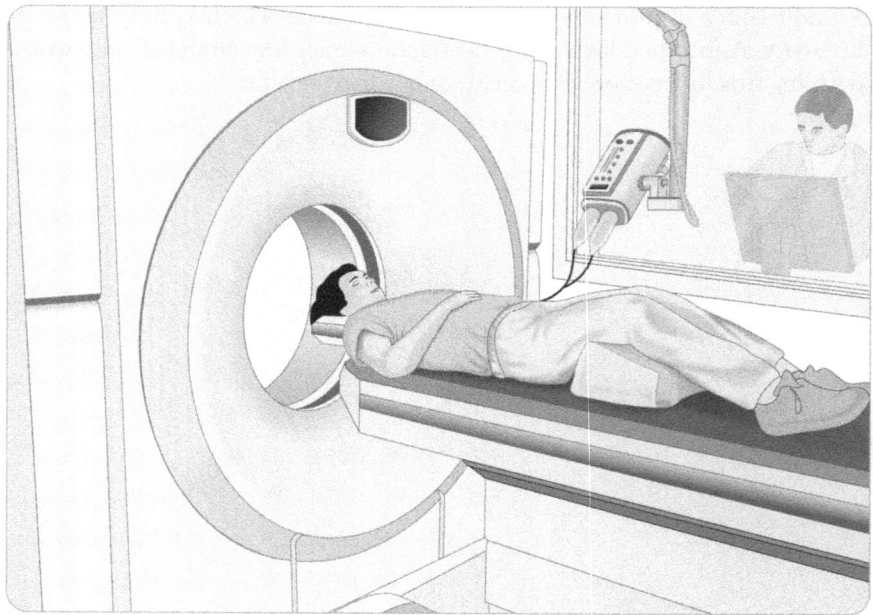

FIG. 1: Magnetic resonance imaging for neurological findings.

arterial dissections, infarcts, cerebral venous thrombosis (CVT), vasculitis, cerebral vasospasm, and subdural or epidural hematomas
- Neoplasms, meningeal metastases, and pituitary tumors
- Cervicomedullary lesions such as Chiari malformations and foramen magnum tumors
- Infections—paranasal sinusitis, meningoencephalitis, cerebritis, and abscess
- Low cerebrospinal fluid pressure syndrome

CHAPTER 8

Primary Headaches

A knowledge about the features of the various types of primary headaches is essential in order to diagnose them and differentiate these headaches from those due to structural causes which are called secondary headaches.

The common types of primary headaches are (Fig. 1):
- Tension-type headaches
- Migraine headaches
- Trigeminal autonomic cephalalgias (TACs)

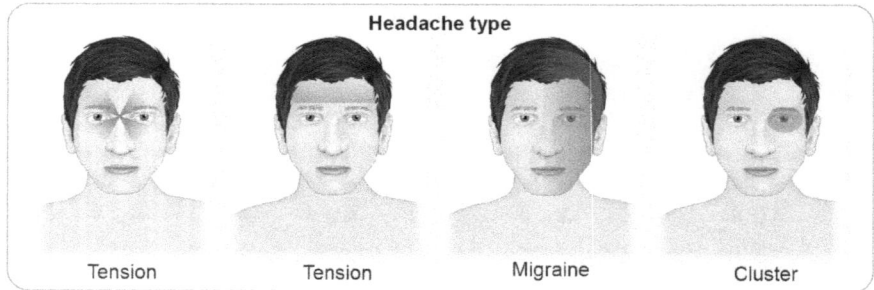

FIG. 1: Sites of various primary headaches.

CHAPTER 9

Migraine

Migraine can be classified into migraine without aura and migraine with aura.

Diagnostic criteria for migraine without aura are:
- Recurrent attacks of at least five attacks of 4–72 hours duration (untreated or unsuccessfully treated)
- The headache has at least two of the following four characteristics:
  1. Unilateral location
  2. Pulsating quality
  3. Moderate or severe pain intensity
  4. Aggravation by or necessitating avoidance of routine physical activity (e.g., walking or climbing stairs)

The headache should be associated with at least one of the following:
- Nausea and/or vomiting
- Photophobia
- Phonophobia

Triggers—sunlight, stress, sleep deprivation, head bath, awakening from sleep, travel, change of weather, hunger, strong odors, hormones, food stuffs, and exercise are the usual triggers of migraine headache.

Diagnostic criteria for migraine with aura are:
- Features of migraine, which are mentioned earlier, associated with fully reversible aura of unilateral visual, retinal, sensory, motor symptoms, or rarely speech disturbance.
- These auras usually last for 5–60 minutes.

CHAPTER 10

Phases of Migraine

Prodrome or premonitory phase could precede the headache by hours to 2 days and consists of changes in mental state, photophobia and/or phonophobia, yawning, drowsiness, and general symptoms such as stiff neck, craving for food, and altered bowel symptoms. Aura phase occurs in about 30% as stated earlier with headache though not necessarily in all. In resolution phase, postdrome symptoms such as changes in mood, weakness/tiredness, anorexia, irritability, and poor concentration could occur **(Fig. 1)**.

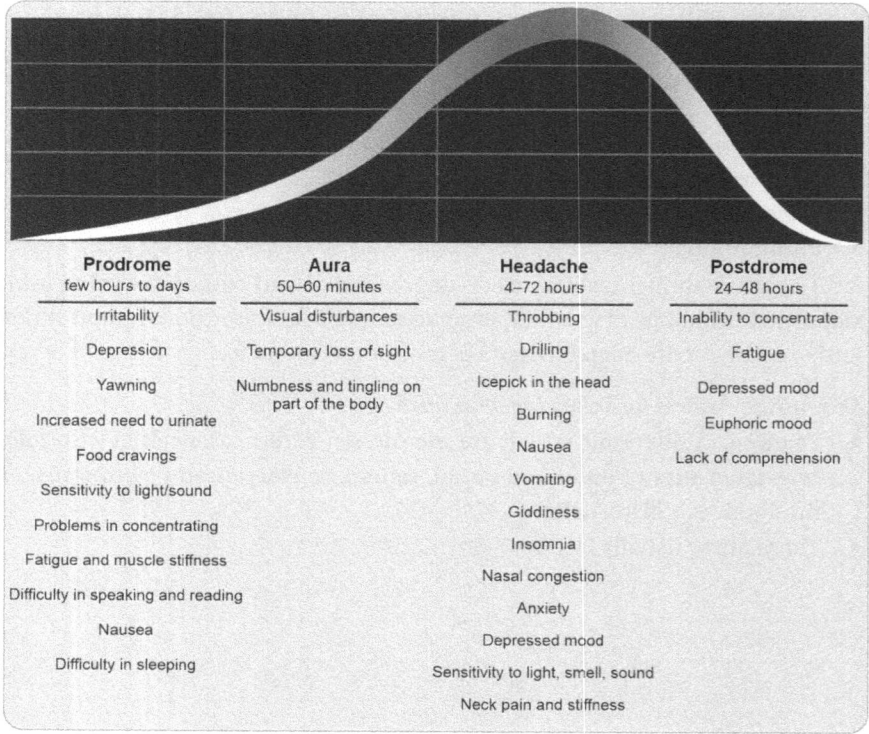

FIG. 1: Timeline of a migraine attack.

CHAPTER **11**

Migraine Features

- Pain in any part of the head or face including upper and lower jaw, teeth, and malar eminence
- It can be unilateral in about 60% or bilateral in 40%.
- In about 15%, the pain is always one sided.
- Migraine which lasts for >72 hours is called status migrainosus.
- If not treated, 80% have fairly severe pain with nausea and the phobias (photo, phono, and osmo)
- Cranial autonomic symptoms of forehead sweating, lacrimation, and nasal congestion could occur though not necessarily during each attack.
- About 70% of migraineurs have a family history of a first-degree relative being affected with similar headaches.

CHAPTER 12

Pathophysiology of Migraine

The following are postulated as the mechanisms of causation of migraine:
- Brainstem neuronal hyperexcitability
- Cortical spreading depression in migraine with aura
- Abnormalities of 5-hydroxytryptophan (5-HTP), calcitonin gene-related peptide (CGRP), norepinephrine (NE), dopamine (DA), gamma-aminobutyric acid (GABA), nitric oxide (NO), glutamate, and endorphins
- Trigeminal activation resulting in dilatation of meningeal vessels (throbbing), activation of area postrema causing nausea and vomiting, activation of cortex and thalamus, resulting in pain over the head, and activation of cervical trigeminal system producing cervical muscle spasm **(Fig. 1)**.

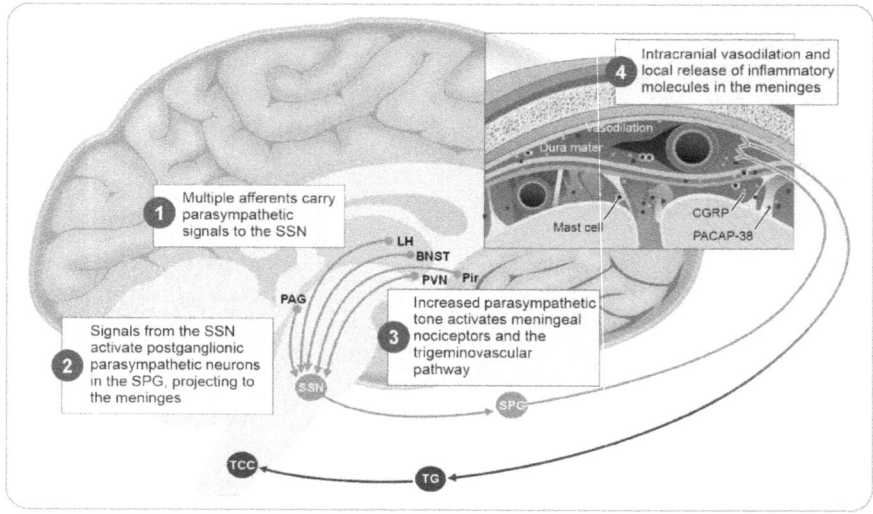

FIG. 1: Activation of meningeal nociceptors by increased parasympathetic tone.

(BNST: bed nucleus of stria terminalis; LH: lateral hypothalamus; PAG: periaqueductal gray; Pir: piriform cortex; PVN: paraventricular hypothalamic nucleus; SPG: sphenopalatine ganglion; SSN: superior salivatory nucleus; TCC: trigeminal cervical complex; TG: trigeminal ganglion)

CHAPTER **13**

Treatment of Migraine

TREATMENT

Medicines for acute treatment and relief of headache:
- Acetaminophen and paracetamol
- Nonsteroidal anti-inflammatory drugs (NSAIDs)—ibuprofen, naproxen sodium, and diclofenac
- Ergotamine not widely used because of adverse effect but is making a comeback
- Triptans—5-hydroxytryptophan 1B (5-HT1B) and 1D receptor agonists. 5-HT1B receptor agonists have a vasoconstricting effect.

Triptans are at present considered to be the most potent medicine for acute treatment by aborting the headache.

Sumatriptan is the most widely used triptan and is available as tablets and injection and nasal spray with least side effect among the triptan and is given as 50 and 100 mg tablets or 50 mg subcutaneous (SC) injection.

Triptans are preferably given once in 24 hours and is limited to use of two to three times per week. However, those who fail to respond to one triptan can be tried on another.

Limitation of Triptans

5-hydroxytryptophan 1B agonists are to be avoided in individuals with coronary artery disease, peripheral vascular disease, cerebrovascular disease, heart blocks, and uncontrolled hypertension in view of its vasoconstricting effect.

5-hydroxytryptophan 1F receptor agonists have been developed and categorized as a new class of triptans—the ditans and lasmiditan are second-line treatment option in those where triptan has failed or a first-line option in person with earlier mentioned risk factors as it does not cause constriction of the blood vessels.

Calcitonin gene-related peptides (CGRPs) antagonists are the newer molecules in the treatment of migraine.

Gepants are a class of medicines in this group, which inhibit the CGRP receptor, and ubrogepant, rimegepant, and atogepant have been approved by the Food and Drug Administration (FDA) in 2019, 2020, and 2021. Real world data of its efficacy and safety are awaited.

The other class of CGRP antagonists is monoclonal antibody, which is useful for prevention of migraine headaches.

CHAPTER **14**

Migraine Prevention

Drugs recommended and established as effective for migraine prophylaxis are:
- Divalproex/sodium valproate 400–1,000 mg/day
- Metoprolol 47.5–200 mg
- Propranolol 120–240 mg
- Topiramate 25–200 mg
- Flunarizine 5–10 mg [not yet approved by the Food and Drug Administration (FDA)]

CHAPTER 15

Tension-type Headaches

- Tension-type headaches (TTHs) are probably the most commonly diagnosed type of headache in family practice.
- TTHs are recurrent episodes of headache lasting 30 minutes to 1 week.
- The headaches are typically bilateral, mild-to-moderate in intensity, nonthrobbing, and are described as dull, pressure like a tight cap or band without associated nausea or vomit but could have either photo- or phonophobia.
- Physical activity has no influence on the headache intensity in the majority and this feature helps differentiating it from migraine.
- The exact cause of TTH remains elusive; pericranial myofascial mechanisms are probably of importance and sensitization of pain *pathways in the central nervous system (CNS) from prolonged nociceptive* stimuli seems responsible for conversion of episodic to chronic TTH.
- It is the least distinct of all headache types though present in 75% of population-based studies.
- The clinical diagnosis is based chiefly on negative features and many secondary headaches may mimic TTH.
- Atypical history or abnormal clinical examination would suggest the need for imaging; however, the vast majority with typical history and normal examination do not need further investigation.
- Differentiating chronic TTH from chronic migraine may be difficult at times, as the features could overlap and many a time both can coexist. *The mnemonic POUND helps separate migraine from TTH.*

    P—pulsatile quality; *O*—duration of 4–72 hours; *U*—being unilateral; *N*—nausea being associated; *D*—disabling intensity of pain.

CHAPTER **16**

Treatment of Tension-type Headache

- Treatment can be divided into pharmacological and nonpharmacological.
- Most persons with infrequent tension-type headache (TTH) might take self-administered over-the-counter (OTC) analgesics.
- For those with frequent episodic TTH, simple analgesics and nonsteroidal anti-inflammatory drugs (NSAIDs) are the mainstays in acute therapy.
- Tricyclic antidepressants (TCAs) are effective for chronic TTH and another option is mirtazapine, a serotonergic and noradrenergic antidepressant.
- The role of muscle relaxants in prevention of chronic TTH is debatable. Centrally acting muscle relaxant like tizanidine may have some benefits.
- Botulinum toxin is not recommended for chronic TTH.
- Nonpharmacological management includes physical therapy, biofeedback, lifestyle changes, and psychological treatment.

CHAPTER 17

Trigeminal Autonomic Cephalgias

- Trigeminal autonomic cephalgias (TACs) are a group of primary headache disorders with pain and/or autonomic features in the distribution of trigeminal nerve.
- The TACs include cluster headache (CH), paroxysmal hemicrania (PH), hemicrania continua (HC), and short-lasting unilateral neuralgiform headache attacks with conjunctival injection and tearing (SUNCT), and short-lasting unilateral neuralgiform attacks with cranial autonomic symptoms (SUNA) but without tearing **(Fig. 1)**.
- The TACs are uncommon, but are disabling and have a major impact on the patient's quality of life.
- These headache disorders are eminently treatable with highly selective drugs that are generally not used for migraine or tension-type headache (TTH).
- Misdiagnosis is common and there could be a delay of several years before the correct diagnosis is made.
- The TACs consist of severe headache attacks accompanied by prominent oculocephalic autonomic features ipsilateral to the headache.
- The general diagnostic characteristics of this group are unilateral head pain predominantly affecting the ophthalmic division of the trigeminal nerve associated with cranial autonomic symptoms with increased parasympathetic and decreased sympathetic activity.
- Human functional imaging studies show activation of trigeminal parasympathetic reflex with secondary cranial sympathetic dysfunction.
- Neuroimaging studies have shown hypothalamic activation ipsilateral to the pain in CH; ipsilateral, contralateral, bilateral, or absent in SUNCT; contralateral in PH and contralateral posterior hypothalamus and ipsilateral dorsal rostral pons in HC.
- CH, PH, and SUNCT can be differentiated from each other based on the duration and frequency of attacks and the therapeutic response.

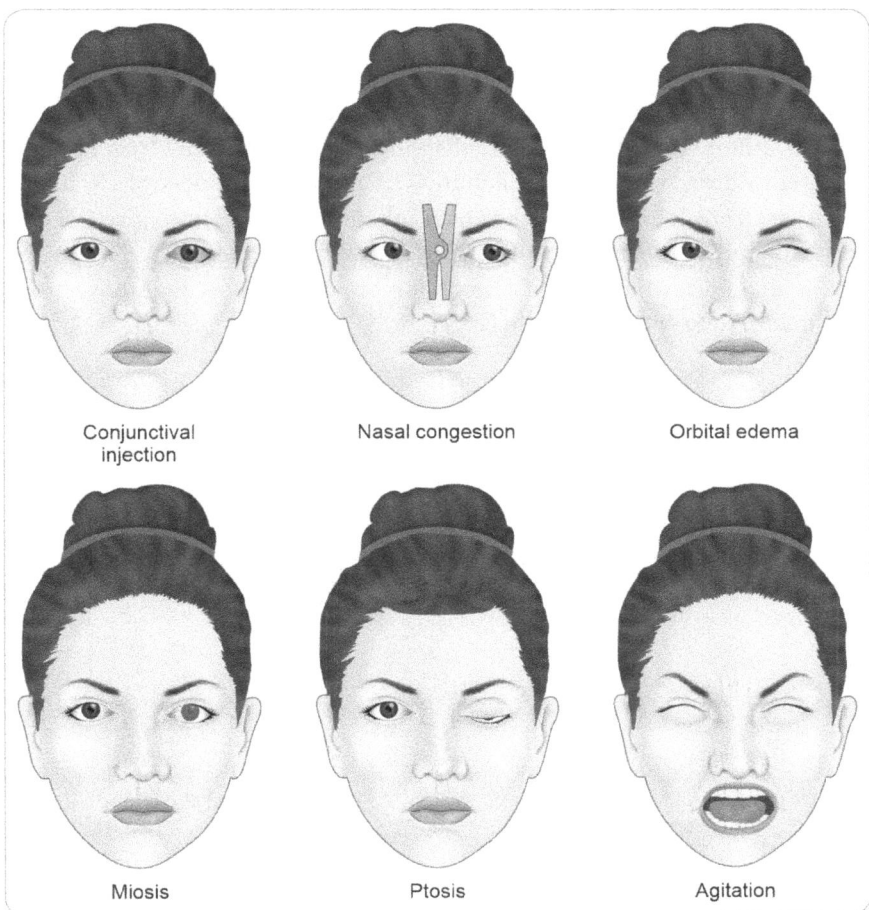

FIG. 1: Trigeminal autonomic symptoms.

- However, there may be an overlap among these three in duration and frequency, and hence, other aspects of these entities need to be considered.
- PH differs from CH mainly in the high frequency and shorter duration of each attack and also by the lack of periodicity and clustering which are seen in CHs.
- SUNCT and SUNA are relatively rare TACs which mimic trigeminal neuralgia in duration but are easily differentiated by the associated prominent autonomic features and resistance to carbamazepine.
- HC is differentiated from other TACs by being unilateral with a continuous moderate intensity pain, which gets accentuated. The history of background continuous pain is vital for the diagnosis.

TREATMENT

- A successful response to O_2 indicates a diagnosis of CH and a positive response to indomethacin is characteristic of PH and HC.
- The indomethacin test can be a diagnostic trial to confirm PH and HC and is considered negative only if there is no response to a dose of 150 mg.
- Apart from 100% O_2, triptans given subcutaneous (SC) can give freedom from pain in the majority of persons with CH.
- Verapamil is the drug of choice for prevention and may have to be increased to 480 mg a day in CH.

CHAPTER **18**

Other Primary Headaches

PRIMARY THUNDERCLAP HEADACHE

- A severe headache of sudden onset reaching maximum intensity in less than a minute is called a thunderclap headache.
- However, a secondary cause of such a headache must be excluded, especially that of subarachnoid hemorrhage (SAH), which could be a cause in 25%, before concluding that this headache is primary.
- Reversible cerebral vasoconstriction syndrome (RCVS), cervical artery dissection, spontaneous intracranial hypotension, and cerebral venous thrombosis are other causes which need to be considered and excluded in persons with a sudden onset, severe headache.

Primary Headache Associated with Sexual Activity

- Sexual activity could produce a bilaterally diffuse or occipital headache lasting from 1 minute to 24 hours of severe intensity, which can be preorgasmic or orgasmic.
- Orgasmic headache could be explosive in onset like a thunderclap and is followed by a severe generalized headache.
- The lifetime prevalence is about 1%.
- Secondary causes mentioned earlier for thunderclap headache need to be excluded and 5% of aneurysmal SAH can occur during sex in 5%.
- Triptans are effective, and can be taken prior to sexual activity or also after occurrence for relief if not taken earlier. Indomethacin and topiramate can also be taken for prevention.

PRIMARY EXERCISE HEADACHE

- Typically a bilateral throbbing headache lasting from minutes to hours related to sustained physical exercise and usually not associated with nausea or vomiting is considered to be a primary exercise-induced headache.

- Occurs in about 10% of the population usually in the age range of 20–40 years.
- Secondary pathology such as space-occupying lesions (SOLs) and vascular abnormalities should be excluded.
- Indomethacin, propranolol, and naproxen can be used for prevention.

HYPNIC HEADACHE

- This is a rare type of headache that occurs only during sleep and awakens the sufferer at a consistent time usually between 1 and 4 AM and can occur during daytime naps also.
- It is not accompanied by nausea or autonomic symptoms and can be unilateral or bilateral, throbbing or nonthrobbing, and can be mild or severe in intensity.
- The duration can range from minutes to hours and can occur frequently but is usually once in a day.
- Usually occurs in persons over 50 years and more often in females.
- The best treatment is caffeine taken before going to sleep apart from lithium and indomethacin.

NEW DAILY PERSISTENT HEADACHE

- New daily persistent headache (NDPH) is a rare, idiopathic, persistent headache with a continuous, unremitting headache with a pinpointed onset and lasting for >3 months.
- The headache is usually bilateral ranging from mild-to-severe and is present in any head region.
- The age of onset ranges from 6 to 70 years and is usually preceded by stress, infection, and surgery.
- NDPH is a diagnosis of exclusion after excluding a host of differential diagnosis such as SOL, spontaneous intracranial hypotension, and idiopathic intracranial hypertension, RCVS, cervical artery dissection, cerebral venous thrombosis, arteriovenous malformation, sinusitis, meningitis, Chiari malformation, and temporal arteritis.
- The headache is treated like migraine or TTH, which it resembles.

NUMMULAR HEADACHE

- It is a recently described circumscribed head pain of mild-to-moderate intensity and is pressure like in nature with a remitting or chronic course.
- It is a primary headache with no underlying lesion usually demonstrated.

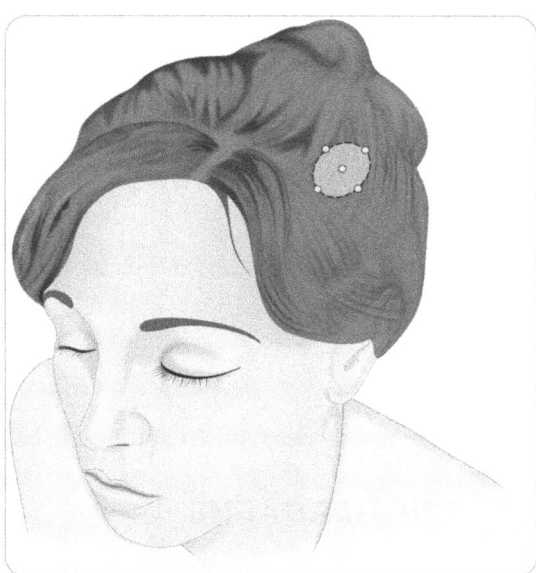

FIG. 1: Site of nummular headache.

- It occurs in one precisely localized site in a small rounded area outlined with paresthesia, hyperesthesia, or dysesthesia on the affected area usually in the parietal region.
- The particular topography suggests a probable epicranial source in a few terminal branches of the cutaneous nerves of the scalp.
- Paracetamol would suffice for relief in most patients with this type of headache as it is not frequent **(Fig. 1)**.

CHAPTER **19**

Secondary Headaches

Secondary headaches are headaches with an underlying cause.

POST-TRAUMATIC HEADACHE

- It is quite common after mild traumatic brain injury.
- The onset should be within 7 days of trauma to quantify for a post-traumatic headache (PTH).
- This headache most often resembles migraine or tension-type headache and can also manifest as occipital, supra- or infraorbital neuralgia, or temporomandibular disorder being localized rather than being diffuse or at multiple sites.
- It is a persistent headache reported in 50–75% for 3 months and up to a year in a third of the patients. Noted to persist even up to 25% at 4 years.
- These headaches are treated with medicines as used in for the primary headache which it resembles.

ALCOHOL HANGOVER HEADACHE

- It may be associated with physical symptoms such as anorexia, tremulousness, diarrhea, dizziness, and fatigue; sympathetic symptoms like tachycardia and sweating; cognitive and mood symptoms such as decreased attention and concentration, anxiety, and irritability.
- Typically, it is a throbbing headache occurring on the morning after alcohol consumption and peaks when the blood alcohol concentration (BAC) is zero and continues up to 24 hours.
- More common in mild-to-moderate drinkers and alcohol can also trigger migraine and cluster headache.
- The effects may be decreased by drinking in moderation and sipping slowly, eating greasy foods before taking alcohol, and taking honey in tomato juice and food rich in fructose and by ensuring good sleep.

HIGH ALTITUDE HEADACHE

- Ascent to an altitude above 2,500 meters can produce acute mountain sickness with a bilateral headache of mild or moderate intensity in many, and resolves within 24 hours of descent to < 2,500 meters.
- It can be associated with nausea, photophobia, vertigo, and poor concentration.
- The risk of high altitude headache (HAH) can be reduced with the use of aspirin taken three times at 4 hours interval and 1 hour before ascent, four doses in total. Ibuprofen three times a day starting 6 hours before ascent can also be given.
- Acetazolamide 125 mg every 12 hours starting a day prior to ascent is also effective.
- This headache can be treated with paracetamol, ibuprofen, and antiemetics.

POSTLUMBAR PUNCTURE HEADACHE

- Postdural puncture headaches (PDPH) are typically bilateral frontal, occipital, or generalized throbbing or pressure-like headaches, worse when upright.
- Occurs within 6–72 hours of the procedure and in the majority lasts < 5 days.
- Can be associated with nausea, vomiting, dizziness, neck stiffness, and visual symptoms.
- Younger (18–30 years) age group, female gender, prior chronic or recurrent headaches, and large diameter needle are the risk factors.
- Bed rest, oral caffeine, and normal saline infusion helps. Persistent headaches are treated with blood patch over the site of the dural puncture.

SPONTANEOUS INTRACRANIAL HYPOTENSION OR LOW CEREBROSPINAL FLUID VOLUME HEADACHES

- Spontaneous intracranial hypotension (SIH) results from spontaneous cerebrospinal fluid (CSF) leaks, typically at the spinal level (thoracic) and seldom at skull base level and can occur at all ages.
- The headache occurs while upright and is relieved on lying down and hence can appear or get relieved on change of posture.
- This headache usually has the characteristics of tension-type headache and can evolve into a nonorthostatic chronic daily headache.
- Can also occur as exertional headache, cough headache, acute thunderclap onset, second-half-of-the-day headaches, and intermittent headaches.

SPONTANEOUS INTRACRANIAL HYPOTENSION HEADACHE

- This headache can be associated with neck stiffness or pain, nausea/vomiting, photo/phonophobia, decreased hearing, tinnitus, or a sense of imbalance.
- MRI brain is abnormal in up to 80% and the most common abnormality is diffuse pachymeningeal enhancement.
- The opening pressure of CSF on lumbar puncture is often low but could be normal as well with no specific attributes.
- Treatment is like that of PDPH.

MEDICATION-OVERUSE HEADACHE

- Headache occurring for >15 days a month as a consequence of taking analgesics regularly for >3 months for relief of headache, is termed medication-overuse headache (MOH).
- It is present in 1–2% of persons with migraine or tension-type headache and is diagnosed more often in headache clinics.
- Treatment includes tapering off the over used medications usually analgesics and substituting with preventives.
- Naproxen 500 mg twice daily can be given alone or in combination with tizanidine for relief.

REVERSIBLE CEREBRAL VASOCONSTRICTION SYNDROME

- This syndrome is characterized by multiple thunderclap headaches associated with nausea and vomiting with photophobia as a predominant manifestation.
- It occurs more often in women in the age range of 20–50 years and occurs postpartum or after exposure to vasoactive drugs such as cannabis, selective serotonin reuptake inhibitor (SSRI), triptans, and intravenous immunoglobulin (IVIg).
- The defining feature of reversible cerebral vasoconstriction syndrome (RCVS) is vasoconstriction of cerebral vessels demonstrated on angiography which reverses within 1–3 months.
- Complications include cervical artery dissection, ischemic or hemorrhagic stroke, cortical subarachnoid hemorrhage (SAH), posterior reversible encephalopathy syndrome (PRES), and seizures.
- Nimodipine, nifedipine, and verapamil can be useful, though there are no placebo controlled trials for these medicines.

CHAPTER **20**

Neuralgias

TRIGEMINAL NEURALGIA

The pain is on one side of the face and it should have at least three of the following features to qualify for it to be a trigeminal neuralgia (TN):
- The pain should be paroxysmal and recurrent, lasting for less than a second to 2 minutes.
- It should be severe in intensity.
- It should be electric shock such as, shooting, stabbing, or sharp in quality.
- Usually is precipitated by tactile stimuli such as washing, toweling, and chewing.
- It should not be associated with a clinical neurological deficit.
- It usually occurs in the fifth or sixth decade and is quite often caused by compression of the nerve by superior cerebellar artery, though secondary causes such as multiple sclerosis (MS), neoplasms, and basilar artery aneurysm have to be considered.
- The pain is most often in the maxillary division (V_2) of the trigeminal nerve or in the mandibular division (V_3) **(Fig. 1)**.

GLOSSOPHARYNGEAL NEURALGIA

- Glossopharyngeal neuralgia causes severe stabbing pain on one side of the throat near the tonsils with occasional radiation to the ear.
- Lasts from less than a second to 2 minutes.
- Precipitated by swallowing, coughing, talking, or yawning.
- Most have an artery pressing on the nerve as it exits the medulla and travels in the subarachnoid space. Other causes include tumors, MS, Paget's disease, and Sjögren syndrome.
- Most often occurs in the fifth or sixth decade.

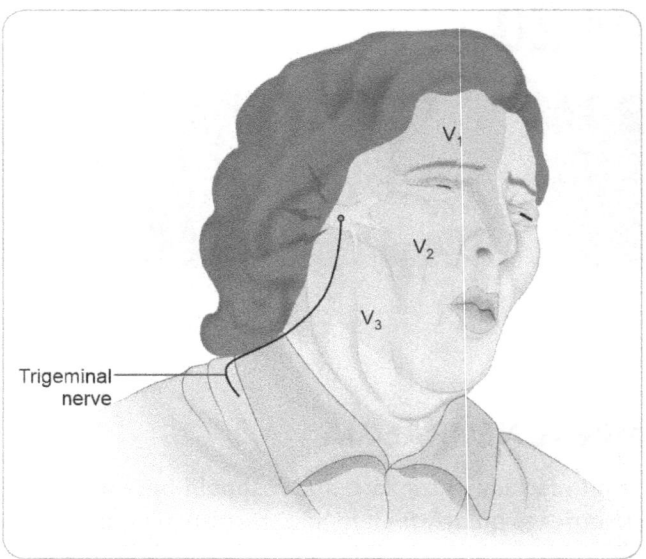

FIG. 1: The distribution of pain in the face according to the branches of the trigeminal nerve causing the pain.

OCCIPITAL NEURALGIA

- The distribution of pain in the face according to the branches of the trigeminal nerve causing the pain.
- It can involve the greater occipital nerve or lesser occipital nerve.
- Paroxysms of electrical pain in the distribution of the nerve and could be referred to suboccipital, hemicranial, temporal, frontal, orbital, periorbital, or retro-orbital distribution.
- Lesser occipital neuralgia occurs over the lateral scalp superior and posterior to the ear and sometimes in the ear.
- Tenderness over the involved nerve can be elicited with reproduction of symptoms.
- Could be associated with hyperesthesia, dysesthesia, or paresthesia over the scalp area.
- Primary and secondary headaches including temporal arteritis can mimic occipital neuralgia.

CHAPTER **21**

Headaches and Sinus Disease

- A widely accepted definition of sinus disease has not been established.
- Inflammation of the sinus is almost always preceded by rhinitis, and hence, the preferred term is rhinosinusitis.
- Acute adult rhinosinusitis is of sudden onset and lasts for up to 4 weeks.
- The examination should include anterior rhinoscopy, otoscopy, and oropharyngeal and neck examinations.
- The task force identified major and minor clinical symptoms and signs for clinical diagnosis. Two or more major factors or one major and two minor factors are essential.

    Major factors:
    - Purulence in nasal cavity
    - Facial pain
    - Nasal obstruction
    - Fever
    - Hyposmia

    Minor factors:
    - Headache
    - Halitosis
    - Fatigue
    - Dental pain
    - Cough
    - Ear pain

- The task force indicated that most cases can be diagnosed clinically.
- Imaging of the sinuses and diagnostic nasal endoscopy is only for difficult cases.
- CT scan is considered as the gold standard for the diagnosis of chronic sinusitis.
- In frontal sinusitis, the headache is directly over the sinus and radiates to the vertex.

- Maxillary sinusitis, the pain is over the antral area radiating to upper teeth or forehead.
- Ethmoidal sinusitis produces pain between and behind the eyes and in sphenoidal sinusitis, the pain is in occipital, vertex, and frontal region **(Fig. 1)**.

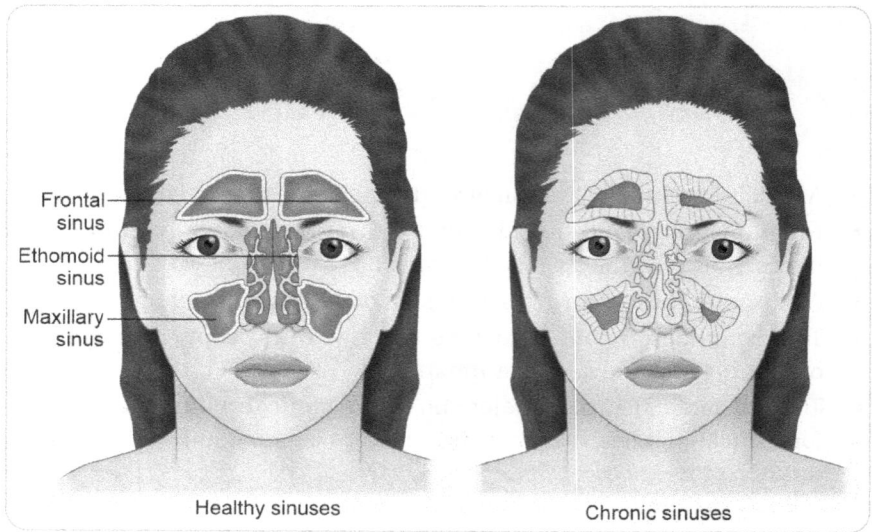

FIG. 1: Types of sinuses.

Note: Headache is considered only as a minor factor for the diagnosis of sinusitis.

CHAPTER **22**

Challenges

WHEN TO INVESTIGATE?

The "red flags" to consider for investigation are:
- Acute or sudden onset of headache or the first or worst headache
- New onset and late onset of headache
- Progressive or worsening headache
- Headache with neurologic symptoms or signs

Secondary headaches could simulate primary headaches or could occur in a person with a preexisting primary headache. Headaches seen in practice may not match with textbook descriptions. There is no investigation protocol that can be used individually for all headache patients, and the investigation has to be customized for each depending on the provisional diagnosis. Misdiagnosis could happen as we attribute all headaches to common conditions such as migraine, hypertension, sinusitis, and cervical spondylosis.

When a person presents with a headache, the first goal should be to find out whether the headache is primary or secondary. This is done based on the description of the headaches outlined earlier. Apart from migraine and tension-type headaches which in its typical presentation can be identified, the other primary headaches may have to be an exclusion diagnosis after excluding an underlying structural cause.

The significant causes which we would need to consider can be grouped for convenience as under:
- Raised intracranial tension—space-occupying lesions such as tumors, hematomas, abscess, granulomas, hydrocephalus, cerebral venous sinus thrombosis, and idiopathic intracranial hypertension. The headaches are usually subacute or chronic and are rather persistent than being episodic. Associated symptoms and focal deficits apart from the sometimes only finding of papilledema would suggest the diagnosis.

- Vascular causes—hemorrhages—subarachnoid hemorrhage (SAH) and intraparenchymal hemorrhage (ICH), infarcts usually in the posterior circulation, vasculitis-like giant cell arteritis (blindness), reversible cerebral vasoconstriction syndrome (RCVS), and cervical arterial dissections (Horner's) are of acute to subacute onset and could be associated with focal deficits and signs as mentioned earlier.
- Infective causes such as meningitis, encephalitis, and granulomas are usually associated with constitutional symptoms of fever, malaise, neck stiffness, and seizures.
- Following trauma, post-traumatic headaches are common and the trauma could de novo cause headache but more often exacerbates or unmasks the underlying migraine or tension-type headache.
- Low pressure headache as in postlumbar puncture and in spontaneous intracranial hypotension (SIH).

CHAPTER **23**

Case Discussion

VIGNETTE 1

A 20-year-old girl came with history of left-sided headache and left half numbness of 3 days duration. The headache peaked within half an hour and was severe and was associated with vomiting. The numbness which was on the entire left half at onset had receded to be faciobrachial of lesser intensity in 2 days.

Even though she had headaches earlier, this was the worst ever headache she had experienced and was associated with numbness. This headache could be considered a thunderclap headache and as she also had numbness very likely there could be an underlying cause. The magnetic resonance imaging (MRI) showed diffusion restriction in the right thalamus corresponding to the numbness on the left side suggestive of ischemia. However, this would not explain adequately the worst ever rapidly peaked headache which she had. The magnetic resonance angiography (MRA) however showed narrowing of the right posterior cerebral artery with irregularities within it which led to the diagnosis of reversible cerebral vasoconstriction syndrome (RCVS).

VIGNETTE 2

Another interesting presentation of RCVS was a 32-year-old lady who had sudden onset of deafness associated with vertigo and vomiting followed by headache was seen by ear, nose, and throat (ENT) surgeon who found no abnormality in the ear and after 2 days treatment had a MRI done which showed blood in one hemispheric sulcus suggestive of subarachnoid hemorrhage (SAH). She improved spontaneously and hence nothing much was done about it. However, she being a young educated, career-oriented lady was anxious to know what happened to her and whether she would regain hearing and what would happen in future. When seen about 3 weeks later for a second neurologic opinion, she had residual hearing loss but no other signs or new symptoms. She, however, continued to have intermittent headaches though not very severe. Ongoing through her initial MRA, vessel irregularity could be seen. She had also had another MRA done because of the SAH to exclude an aneurysm and on this MRA the irregularity was not seen suggesting the possibility of RCVS. The hearing loss and vertigo were because of ischemia in the anterior inferior cerebellar artery (AICA) territory, and she had an independent site SAH, both of which are known features with RCVS.

VIGNETTE 3

A 43-year-old man presented with acute onset pain in the nuchal occipital region on the right side associated with vertigo when he happened to suddenly look up on hearing a noise coming from upstairs. He did not lose consciousness and did not have vomiting but every time he extended the neck he experienced a sharp headache on right side and vertigo. The mode of occurrence and the description of symptoms suggested the possibility of dissection of the neck vessel. He did not have Horner's which would have clinched the diagnosis. He had already had a MRI done which was normal. As the history was rather typical, an MRA was requested asking the radiologist to look out for dissection of a neck vessel and indeed the right vertebral artery showed an intramural dissection.

Management is with anticoagulants followed by antiplatelet agents **(Figs. 1A and B)**.

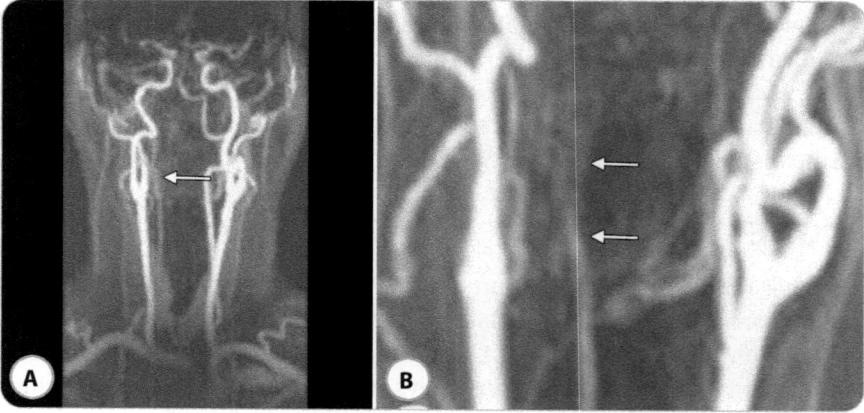

FIGS. 1A AND B: Contrast-enhanced magnetic resonance angiography showing a normal proximal right vertebral artery with irregularities and tapering in the high cervical portion.

VIGNETTE 4

A lady in mid 30s came to the headache clinic with history of headaches, which varied in severity and duration and was intermittent. She had taken treatment with a practitioner with temporary relief. On examination, she had no findings but on re-eliciting the history it became apparent that the headaches occurred only when she was sitting or standing and walking and not while lying down. An MRI was requested because of this history which confirmed the presence of pachymeningitis. She was managed conservatively as spontaneous intracranial hypotension (SIH) with increased fluid intake and amitriptyline with improvement, though headaches do continue to occur less frequently **(Figs. 2A and B)**.

VIGNETTE 5

A young male, 29 years of age, came to the outpatient department (OPD) with history of global headache of about 3 weeks duration with increasing severity but with no associated symptoms. He used to consume alcohol and take more during weekends. He did not show neurological deficit but had papilledema. MRI showed superior sagittal sinus thrombosis, and he was treated with anticoagulants **(Figs. 3A and B)**.

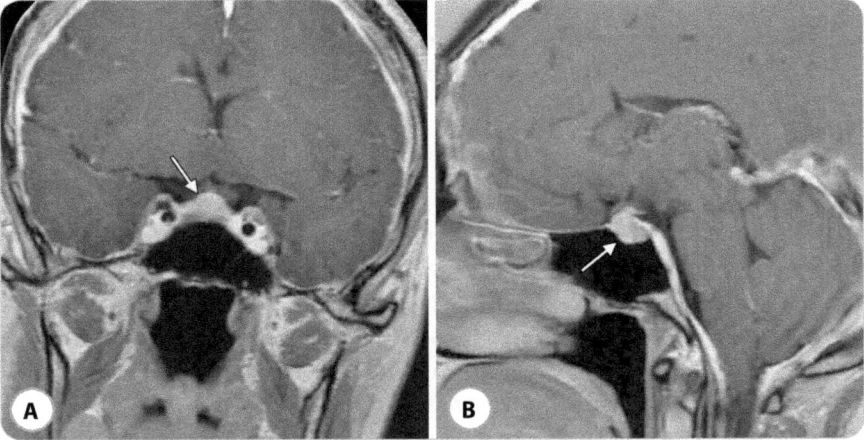

FIGS. 2A AND B: Magnetic resonance examination in patients with intracranial hypotension (IH). T1-weighted post-contrast images: (A) Coronal and (B) sagittal images demonstrate an enlargement of the pituitary gland (arrow) and a significant pachymeningeal enhancement.

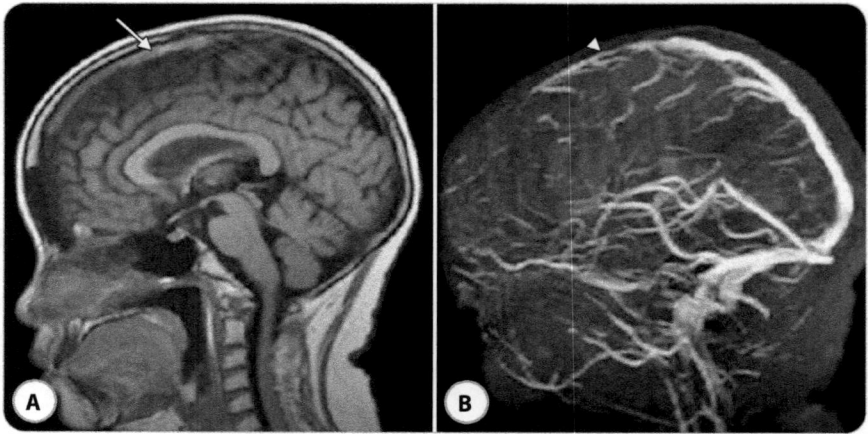

FIGS. 3A AND B: T1-weighted sagittal image showing a hyperintense thrombus (white arrow) within the anterior half of superior sagittal sinus. The thrombus is shown on the 2D-TOF MRV as a focal flow void abnormality (white arrowhead).

(MRV: magnetic resonance venography; TOF: time-of-flight)

VIGNETTE 6

A man in his 60s complained of a nagging but nonsevere headache of close to 2 months duration. The headache had no specific features and the patient was also unable to give further details. The ocular fundi were normal and there was no weakness. However, his right plantar was extensor and a CT scan of the head showed a subdural hemorrhage (SDH), which was subsequently evacuated **(Fig. 4)**.

VIGNETTE 7

A 19-year-old college student, mildly obese, came with history of headaches of close to 6 years duration satisfying the criteria of migraine without aura and responding each time to Saridon. However, the headaches were felt to be more severe in the past 2 months, because she did not take Saridon as advised by her parents. During this period she felt her vision was becoming blurred and hence referred by her family doctor to ophthalmologist who did not find anything abnormal and hence referred to neurologist. She had papilledema in the left eye more than the right and MRI showed widening of perioptic sheath and partial empty sella. She is on treatment as idiopathic intracranial hypertension. Magnetic resonance venography (MRV) has been requested as she refused to have lumber puncture (LP) done on her to check the opening pressure of cerebrospinal fluid (CSF) and thereby confirm the diagnosis of idiopathic intracranial hypertension **(Figs. 5A and B)**.

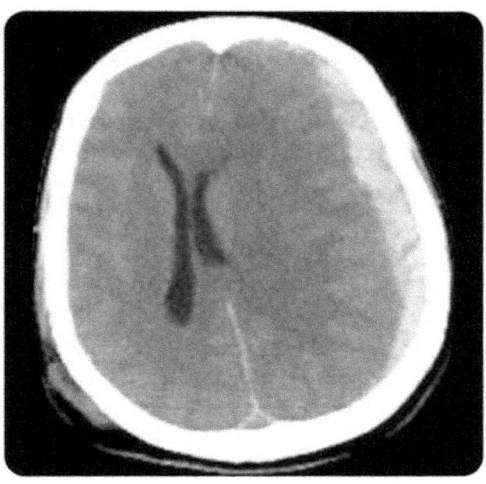

FIG. 4: CT brain showing left-sided subdural hemorrhage (SDH).

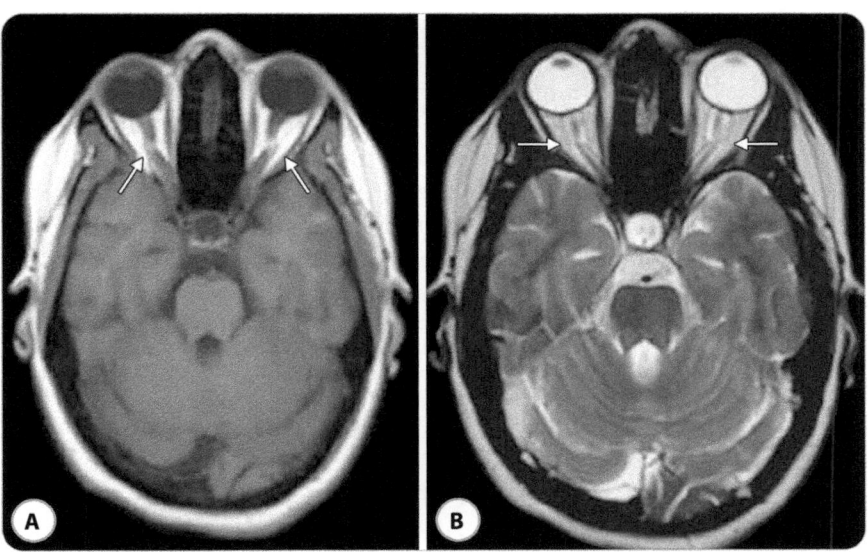

FIGS. 5A AND B: Magnetic resonance imaging of brain. (A) T1-weighted and (B) T2-weighted axial images at the level of optic nerve (ON) reveal bilateral tortuous ON on T1-weighted sequence with prominent cerebrospinal fluid spaces around it on T2-weighted.

VIGNETTE 8

A 63-year-old man had a road traffic accident with a brief period of loss of consciousness and was admitted and observed for 2 days. He had no further symptoms and a CT scan of the head was normal. A week later he had intermittent headaches mostly over the posterior head region and another CT scan was done, which was also normal. However, he continues to have intermittent headaches of a pressing nature and gives history of having had headaches earlier in his 20s and 30s. With treatment as for tension-type headache, he is better and the diagnosis is post-traumatic headache.

VIGNETTE 9

A 65-year-old man presented with a focal area of left temporal headache of 1 year duration. The pain was rather constant with exacerbation and remission depending on analgesic use. For the past 1 year he has been treating himself with aceclofenac and paracetamol 1 tablet in the morning and evening for pain relief and if he does not take the medicine he gets headache which is not associated with nausea or vomiting. It is not associated with autonomic symptoms either. The C-reactive protein (CRP) and erythrocyte sedimentation rate (ESR) were within normal range and MRI was normal.

The differential diagnosis in this patient could be the following:
Nummular headache: The localized small area of pain is in favor and also the lack of other symptoms is in favor of this diagnosis. However, the persistent pain is usually not a feature as it is mostly intermittent. Giant cell arteritis is another differential because of the site, persistence, and the age. However, the ESR and CRP were in the normal range. Hemicrania continua described earlier under primary headache is another possibility but lacks the autonomic component. Localized headache could be secondary to an underlying abnormality, which was excluded by a normal MRI. The provisional diagnosis is medication-overuse headache arrived at by a process of exclusion.

Index

A
Alcohol hangover headache 26
Approach 3
Aura 6

C
CGRP (calcitonin gene related peptide) 14
Cluster headache 20
Cortical spreading depression 14

G
Glossopharyngeal neuralgia 29

H
Hemicrania continua (HC) 20
High altitude headache 27
Hypnic headache 24

M
Magnetic resonance imaging (MRI) 8
Medication-overuse headache 28
Migraine 11

N
New daily persistent headache 24
Nonsteroidal anti-inflammatory drugs (NSAIDs) 15
Nummular headache 24

O
Occipital neuralgia 30

P
Paroxysmal hemicrania (PH) 20
Pathophysiology of migraine 14
Phases of migraine 12
Postlumbar puncture headache 27
Post-traumatic headache 26
Primary headache 10
Prevention 17

R
Reversible cerebral vasoconstriction syndrome (RCVS) 23

S
Secondary headaches 26
SUNCT 20
SUNA 20
SNOOP 7
Spontaneous intracranial hypotension 27

T
Tension type headache 18
Thunderclap headache 23
Trigeminal autonomic cephalalgia (TAC) 20
Trigeminal neuralgia 29
Triptans 15

EU GSPR Authorised Reprsentative
Logos Europe, 9 rue Nicolas Poussin
1700, La Rochelle, France
Phone: +33 (0) 6 67 93 73 78
E-mail: contact@logoseurope.eu

An Overview of
HEADACHES